SOLUTIONS FOR BETTER SLEEP

Improve Sleeping Positions to Relieve Pain and Stiffness

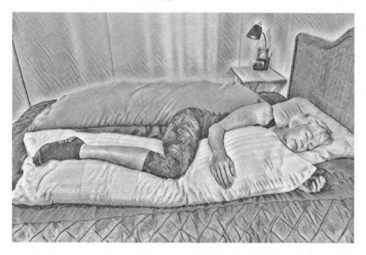

Part of the *Preventing Spinal Sabotage Mayhem, Myths, and Management* Series

Dr. Kathleen M. Favaloro, DC, PT

D1595949

Published by KMF Books.
Printed in the United States of America.
Line drawings by Josiah Branal.
Cover picture illustrated by Viktoriia Davidova.

ISBN# 978-1-956900-06-4 (ebook)
ISBN# 978-1-956900-07-1 (hardback)
ISBN# 978-1-956900-08-8 (paperback)

Thank You for Purchasing
Solutions for Better Sleep!

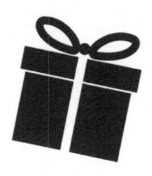

As a thank you gift, I would like to offer you two things to share with your family and friends: a free guide to making your own body pillow, and a free summary of how to transfer in and out of bed safely.

To download your free gifts and for more information about upcoming books, visit KMFbooks.com. I look forward to helping you achieve better sleep and greater spinal health through better positioning!

Sweet dreams,

Dr. Kathleen M. Favaloro, DC, PT

Book Dedication

This book is dedicated to my patients. They are my focus and inspiration, my beloved students and teachers, and my intended audience. I have learned much from them.

They have collectively inspired and motivated me to learn more, try more, do more, and go the extra mile. They touched my heart as I willingly and enthusiastically did my best to help them overcome their challenges, meet their goals, and exceed their expectations.

I empathize with them when they are in pain, and I celebrate with them as the happy smile of understanding and pain relief, at last, returns to their faces.

My goal is to help empower my patients to confidently and successfully handle their day-to-day biomechanical challenges, prevent injury, and enjoy a healthy spine.

It has been an honor and a privilege to share their healing journeys and to witness God's miracles on a daily basis. Thanks to one and all who have accompanied me on this life journey.

Spinal Sabotage

What is spinal sabotage?

Is it some big thing we do to purposely wreck our spine?

Certainly not!

It's the little things:

- Our habits.
- Our postures.
- It's our impulsive or momentary movements.
- It's the unexpected jolts or reflexive grabs, jerks, or jumps.
- It's our exercise programs—or lack of them.
- It's the way we sit, stand, sleep, bend, and carry.
- It's the things we do too much of.
- The things we hardly ever do.
- The things we do every day.

It's the things we least suspect.

Contents

Chapter 1

Introduction to Sleep

How To and How NOT to Sleep:

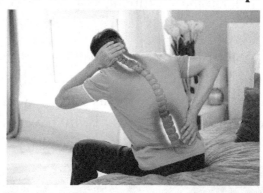

Even sleeping postures can cause injury.

Even though a **good sleep** is typically defined by how long and how deeply we sleep, there is so much more to the story. The better we sleep, the better we think, feel and function when we are awake. Sleep allows the body time to recharge and rejuvenate itself and is essential to good health.

Yet, many patients report that their worst time of day is when they first wake up from sleep and try to get up out of bed. They are stiff, sore, and have difficulty standing up straight. This is often a direct result of the position they slept in. Most people don't realize that improper sleeping positions, especially those that twist and torque the spine, can be dangerous to your health and well-being.

Poor sleeping positions can cause a decrease in blood supply to the brain and reduce nerve function throughout the body, leading to pain and dysfunction, morning stiffness, and even sciatica.

In this book, you will learn several easy ways to optimize your sleeping positions, improve support to your spine and nervous system, and improve your overall health while you sleep.

First, it is important to understand a little bit about the nervous system and why its ability to function optimally is so vital to our health.

Our nervous system has two very distinct parts that, together, govern all of our body's functions, actions, and communication networks. They are known as the sympathetic and parasympathetic nervous systems. Both have billions of tiny neurons that transmit the information necessary for function.

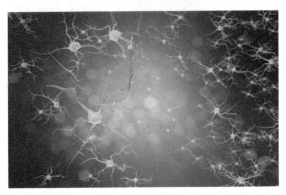

The sympathetic nervous system is in charge of our volitional or voluntary activities. It directs most of our daytime activities, such as the skeletal muscle actions of our arms and legs and our fight, flight, and stress responses.

In contrast, the parasympathetic nervous system mainly supports our internal organ functions and is most active when we sleep. It regulates our homeostasis activities, like repairing and regenerating cells to replace old, worn-out ones, and it makes red blood cells, antibodies, and T cells to strengthen our immune functions.

It also directs the detoxification of the kidneys and liver and purifies the blood and lymph systems. In general, it controls our ability to rest, replenish, digest, and heal.

The parasympathetic nervous system functions best during sleep when our energy is not otherwise diverted and drained by our daily activities like walking, running, and stressing about work. Thus, good quality sleep is essential.

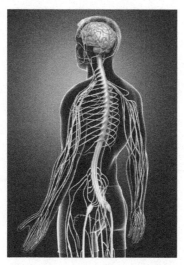

Our nervous system starts in the brain and extends via the spinal cord to the rest of the body. The spinal cord is protected by the boney vertebra that makes up the cervical, thoracic, and lumbar spine.

Sleeping in a biomechanically good position prevents twisting and torquing of the vertebrae and allows the body to relax. It also helps ensure clear and open channels for the spinal cord and nerves to communicate easily with all of their target muscles, organs, and glands.

Twisting and torquing the spine while sleeping can disturb vital nerve pathways, interfere with proper nerve transmission, and cause us to wake up feeling sore, groggy, or out of sorts.

Bad habits and faulty sleeping positions can sabotage the quality of your sleep and your health. Despite the potential for injury, some sleeping habits can be hard to give up, just like any other bad habit or addiction, especially if someone has been doing it for years.

This book will cover "how to" and "how not to" sleep, with pictures and descriptions detailing solutions and alternatives, to improve sleeping habits, optimize the quality of sleep, and improve your health.

Chapter 2

Suffocating Stomach Sleeping

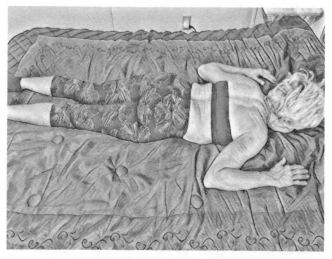

Suffocating Stomach Sleeping

Have you ever been in a sound sleep and, upon awakening, noticed yourself or your children sleeping on their stomachs? Let me ask you: How do they breathe? Of course, people tell me "Through their nose or mouth," ... Ah yes, but what about their spine?

The only way to breathe when sleeping on their stomach without being suffocated by the pillow or the bed is to turn their neck to about 70–90 degrees to one side or the other.

NOTE: Twisting the neck kinks nerves and blood vessels.

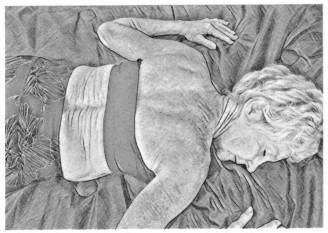

Now a small, hyper-flexible child may get away with that, but in adults, most people don't have that much available rotation, and even if they do—imagine what that does to the nerves and arteries of the neck. They are twisted and often compressed, reducing the blood flow to your brain by up to 60 percent. Additionally, prolonged twisting of the vertebra (whether awake or asleep) can bulge the disc and cause nerve pressure. This can lead to numbness and tingling in your arms and hands, a stiff neck, or back pain.

As a reformed stomach sleeper myself, I totally understand the sense of comfort and security in having something pressed up against and fully supporting your belly. Still, there are other ways to get that same feeling that are much safer for your spine.

Chapter 3

Safer Side Sleeping

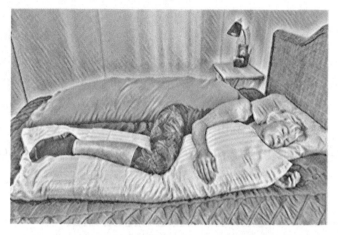

Stomach-Sleeping Solution

The best solution I have found for most people who sleep on their stomach is side sleeping with a long, large "body pillow" pressed against the belly and supporting the top leg and arm. Your body's weight will lean forward toward the pillow, giving the "sense" of stomach sleeping because of the same comforting pressure against your stomach—but without torquing your neck or back.

Side Sleeping with a Body Pillow Can "Feel Like" You Are on Your Stomach.

For Safer Side Sleeping,
Use Proper Pillow Support

Sleeping on your side is generally a good way to sleep, provided you have the right kind of pillow support. In addition to supporting your top arm and leg with a body pillow, like the one on the previous page, there should be a small pillow under your head to take up the space between your shoulder and head. The proper pillow height will vary from person to person. An ideal pillow should support your head in a neutral position to prevent sideways kinking of your neck.

Unsafe Side Sleeping:
Using Improper Pillow Support

Sleeping on your side with too high, too low, or no pillow under your head tilts the head to the side. This causes an awkward side bending and wedging of the vertebrae that can force the disc toward the opposite side's lateral spinal nerve and lead to numbness, tingling, and pain down the arm. It can also cause compensatory spinal twisting in the middle and lower back and lead to sciatica or reduced nerve supply to the heart or lungs.

Kinking the neck without a pillow:
Notice how the head drops.

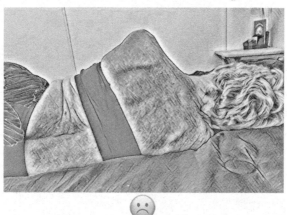

Kinking the neck with TOO HIGH a pillow:
Notice both the neck and spinal twist.

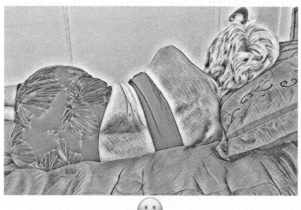

Review: If you wake up in the morning with back pain, a stiff neck, or numbness and tingling in your hands, first, be sure you are not sleeping on your stomach. Then, check the height of your pillow.

Proper Pillow Support
for the Top Leg and Arm

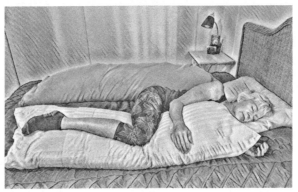

A body pillow is one of the best ways to properly support your top arm and leg and protect your spine when sleeping on your side. For optimum support, be sure the pillow is long enough to extend from your upper chest to the shin of your bottom leg. In addition, the pillow should be wide enough (front to back), plump enough (bottom to top), and firm enough to allow your upper leg and arm to be level and comfortable when resting on the pillow.

If the body pillow is the correct thickness, it will keep the leg parallel to the bed and prevent the knee or foot from tipping up or down, and it will be large enough and stable enough to allow the top leg to easily stay on the pillow, even as the leg bends or straightens. It will also keep you off your stomach.

Torquing the Spine
with No Pillow Support

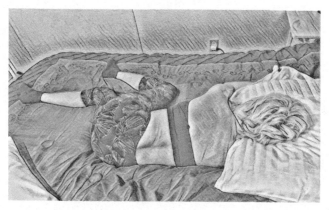

Notice the spinal twist.

When sleeping on your side without a pillow to properly support your top leg and arm, the resultant upper and lower spine twisting and torquing can lead to morning stiffness, pain and even sciatica. It will be also be easier to flop onto your stomach and reduce the blood and nerve supply to the brain.

Torquing the Spine
with Pillows Between the Legs

Putting a pillow BETWEEN the legs isn't much better than no pillow at all because the upper body can still twist forward. Plus, in order to successfully keep the pillow between the legs and prevent the top leg from falling off the pillow, not only do the legs have to be lined up, one on top of the other, they must remain fairly bent all night long.

Torquing the Spine
with Pillows BETWEEN the legs

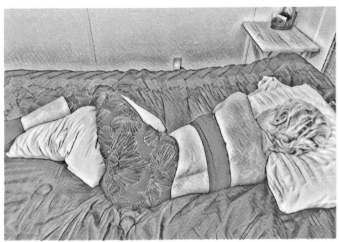

Note the bent hips and knees and spinal twist.

The bent position (pictured above) prevents the hamstring muscles in the back of the thigh and the psoas muscles in the abdomen from stretching out. The main function of the hamstrings is to bend the knees, and because they attach to the lower pelvis, they can also bring the thigh backward. If the hamstrings get too tight, it can lead to sciatica.

The psoas muscles bring the belly and the thighs together. When they get too tight from sitting all day, or from being bent up toward the chest all night, it makes it harder to stand up straight, especially first thing in the morning.

Torquing the Spine More
When the Leg Falls off the pillow

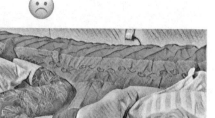

Unfortunately, as hard as one might try to keep the pillow balanced between the legs, the top leg can easily fall off the pillow as the legs move about during the night.

Solution for Spinal Torquing:
Safe Side Sleeping

To prevent spinal torquing and twisting, and tightening of the hamstring and psoas muscles when sleeping on your side, place a long body pillow beside your belly extending from your upper chest to the shin of your bottom leg. Then place your uppermost leg and arm on top of the pillow so they are supported in a level and comfortable position.

Safe Side Sleeping

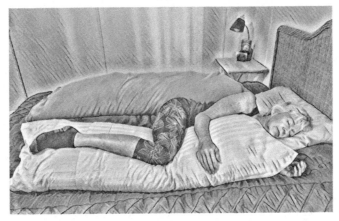

The top arm and leg are supported and level.

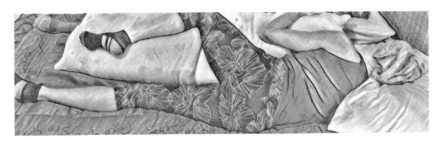

The bottom leg is straight and behind the pillow:
Note the spine is straight and not twisted.

Make sure that your pillow is on the bed directly in front of your straight bottom leg (not on top of it). Also, be sure that your chest and belly, as well as your bottom leg, are in contact with the back of the pillow.

Body Pillow Review:

Sleeping on your side with a body pillow helps keep your spine well-aligned by supporting your top leg and arm in a level, comfortable position. This helps prevent your spine from twisting and allows your back and bottom leg muscles to relax in a straight position.

Using a proper-sized body pillow will keep you off your stomach and thus, help optimize the blood and nerve supply to your brain.

Because this position allows your bottom leg's hamstring and psoas muscles to stretch out, it makes standing up straighter in the morning a lot more likely.

Note: Be sure when you roll to face the other direction, there is another body pillow waiting for you to land on. This way, the other leg also gets a chance to stretch out. 🙂

Remember: You can either purchase a body pillow OR you can make your own.

(Download your free guide on how to make your own body pillow at KMFbooks.com.)

Chapter 4

Better Back Sleeping

Some people believe that sleeping on your back is the best way to sleep. That depends. For some, especially those with a CPAP machine or with a long leg cast on, it may be one of the easier positions to sleep in. Nonetheless, there is a right way and a wrong way to sleep on your back.

Wrong Ways to Sleep on Your Back:

1) Fat pillows kink the neck and bulge the disc.

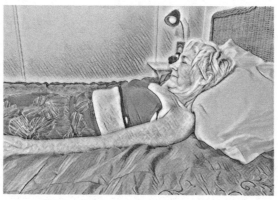

Sleeping on your back with a fat pillow under your head will force the head into a forward flexed position that can bring the fronts of the vertebrae together, like biting the front of the ice cream sandwich. This position kinks the neck and pushes the vulnerable gelatinous disc backward, bulging it out toward the spinal cord. It results in poor posture, stiff neck, and pain and dysfunction of the arms and the neck.

2) Pillows under the knees lead to tight muscles and poor posture.

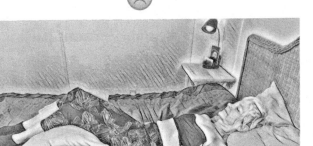

Sleeping on your back with a pillow under your knees is also a common mistake. Though it may give temporary comfort in an acute low back pain episode by taking some pressure off the lower back, it prevents the hamstring and psoas muscles from fully lengthening.

Over time, if the hamstring and psoas muscles do not fully lengthen, they get tighter and shorter, making it more difficult for the knees and back to fully straighten when standing or walking. The resultant forward bent posture will bring the fronts of the vertebrae together, forcing the discs to bulge backward toward the spinal cord, leading to sciatica, difficulty walking, and pervasive pain and dysfunction, especially of the legs and the back.

Back Sleeping Solution

If you wish to sleep on your back, use a very thin pillow or no pillow under your head to prevent your head from bending up and forward. Also, do NOT use a pillow under your knees. Lie flat to allow your hamstring and psoas muscles to lengthen and stretch out. In this position, your entire spine can also lengthen and relax. Ideally, your arms should rest beside you, not up over your head.

Better Back Sleeping: NO pillows.

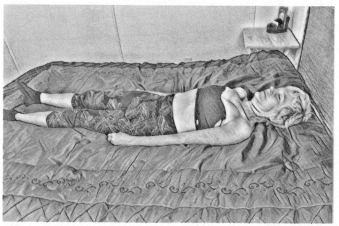

Lie flat, straight, and fully lengthened.

Note: Many people start out on their back but inadvertently end up on their side (or stomach). To prevent the consequences of sleeping in positions that can sabotage your body mechanics and spinal health, it is good to review the principles of Safer Side Sleeping and to be prepared with a body pillow on either side of you. This is very important because most people, regardless of their good intentions, do NOT stay in one position all night long.

Safe, Comfortable Side Sleeping with Proper Pillow Support

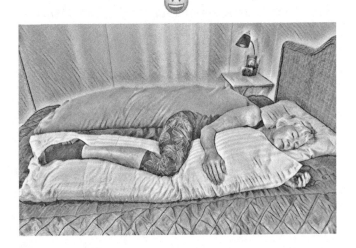

Note: There is also a pillow behind the person, so when they roll over, their top leg will be always be supported, and their spine will stay straight.

Safe, Comfortable Side Sleeping with Pillows

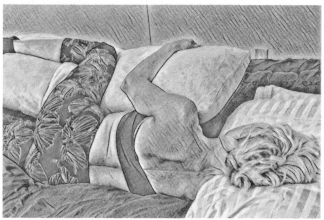

The spine is straight; the top arm and leg are supported.

In this picture, notice how well-supported the top arm and leg are and how straight the spine is. This will allow maximum relaxation with the least amount of spinal stress and torque. If the head pillow is not too fat, the person will be able to use it to support their neck when they lie on their back too.

Chapter 5

Sleeping with Others

What about sleeping with someone else? When another person is sharing your bed, a proper sleeping position for both of you is essential. There are various ways, even in a small bed, to accomplish this.

OPTION 1) When cuddle time is over, and it is time to sleep, place a shared pillow between you and your bedmate to support your top legs when facing each other. When facing the outer edge of the bed, be sure you each have your own cuddle body pillow to support your upper arm and leg and prevent spinal torquing.

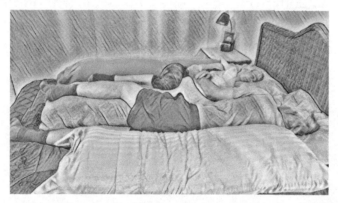

Note the pillows on both sides and in the middle.

Sharing a Center Pillow

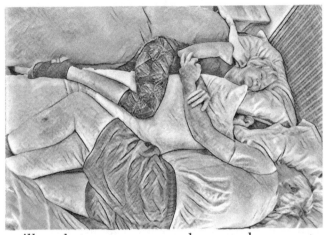

Placing a pillow between you and your sleep mate can also protect you both from being kicked or scratched during restless leg syndrome episodes.

You have choices: Center pillow or side pillow.

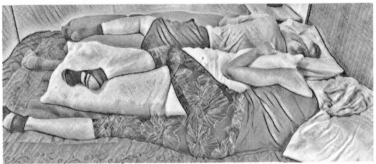

Using multiple pillows ensures support on either side.

OPTION 2) Even in smaller beds, it is still important to have a pillow on each edge to catch the top leg and arm when facing outward. When facing your bedmate, in beds with no space for a center pillow, place your top leg and arm on your bedmate or their side cuddle pillow, as seen in this picture. And when your bedmate faces you, their leg will rest on yours.

Sharing a Side Pillow in Small Beds

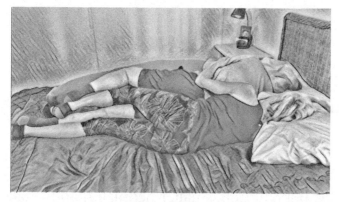

Note: The woman's side cuddle pillow is not shown in this picture, so her leg position could be visible.

Side Pillows For Small Beds

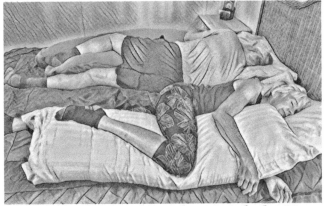

These can be shared or used alone.

Caution: Sleeping with Children and Pets

Larger bedmates and big dogs may be able to support the weight of your leg, but children, smaller bedmates, and small pets may not. So, as you carefully try to avoid landing on their little bodies, please be mindful of your own spinal posture as well as their safety. Compromising your sleeping position, regardless of the reason, will put you at risk for spinal torquing, pain, and stiffness.

In many cases, kids and small pets do better in their own beds. If they are rambunctious, restless, or twitchy sleepers, you may find that you, too, sleep better without those disturbances to your own sleep cycle.

Chapter 6

Dangers of Reading in Bed

Many people lull themselves to sleep with a good book. However, when reading in bed, it is very important to be mindful of the position of your neck when doing so. Looking down at a book on your lap while sitting upright in bed or in a chair, or bunching pillows under your neck to more easily look down at your book, will cause forward wedging of the vertebrae and backward migration of the disc toward the spinal cord. The closer the disc slides and bulges toward the spinal cord, the more likely there will be nerve pressure on the delicate spinal cord or its nerve roots, resulting in pain and dysfunction.

Note the terribly bent neck.

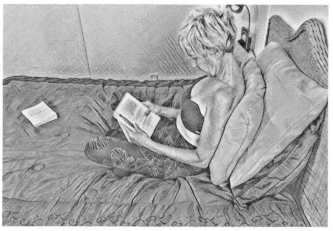

Typically, this isn't something that happens the first time or even the first few times you do it. It happens over time, little by little, by little. Then one day, the disc gets so far back that the next little sneeze, jerk, or the tip down of the head causes sudden and intense pain. When that happens, people tend to attribute it to the final movement or activity that happened just before the traumatic pain began, instead of attributing it to the repeated and gradual, low-intensity assaults that finally added up to the proverbial and inevitable final "straw that broke the camel's back."

A bent neck and rounded shoulders lead to poor posture and spinal kinking.

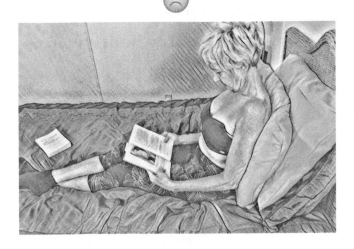

Reading in Bed Solution

If you insist on reading "in" bed, then I highly recommend that you lie flat on your back, without a pillow under your head, and with your knees straight or bent. Place some pillows on your belly and prop your arms or your elbows on the pillows. Put the book in your hands and bend your elbows until the book comes perfectly into view.

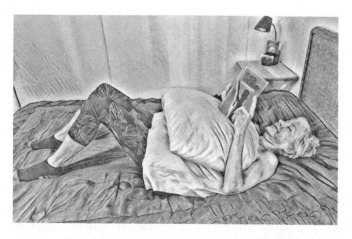

Proper reading in bed: Lie flat with legs up or down and arms supported.

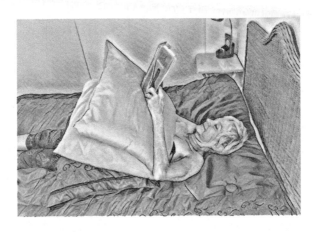

When you get tired, you can put the book down and grab one small pillow for under your neck. Then grab your two body pillows and place one on either side of you. This way, whichever side you turn to will already have a nicely positioned body pillow to catch and support your top leg and arm while you sleep. They will act as soft fluffy guardians that prevent you from rolling onto your stomach or twisting your lower back or pelvis.

Try NOT to fall asleep on your back with pillows under your knees. Doing so would force your knees to stay bent all night long. Any position that prevents your knees and hamstrings from stretching out can lead to tight hamstrings, a precursor to sciatica.

Now that you know how to position yourself while you are in bed, let's talk about how to get into and out of bed safely.

Note: The next section is a bonus. It's an excerpt from my next book about preventing spinal sabotage. I added it to help improve the body mechanics of the spine while getting in and out of bed, as those are times when the spine can easily get torqued and even injured. It can lead to pain, dysfunction, and even disc bulging when done wrong. A summary of safe ways to get into and out of bed located at the end of the next two chapters can be downloaded at KMFbooks.com.

Chapter 7

Safe Ways to Get into Bed

Part A. Going from standing to sitting: Steps 1-2.

<u>Step 1.</u> Walk up to the bed and touch the side of one thigh to the mattress. Then turn backward until the back of both thighs are touching the edge of the bed.

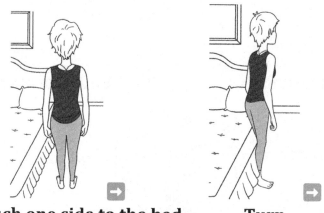

Touch one side to the bed. **Turn.**

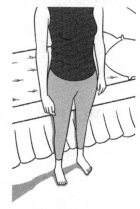

Touch the bed with the back of both legs.

Step 2. Reach back with both hands and push your buttocks backward toward the bed. Your waist and knees will bend. Continue until you are firmly seated on the bed.

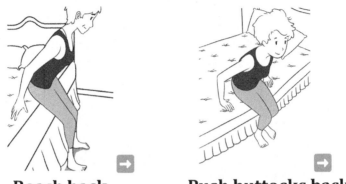

Reach back. 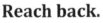 **Push buttocks back.**

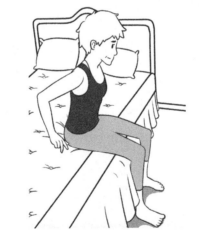

Lower until firmly seated.

Part B. Reclining from sitting to side-lying: Steps 3–4.

Step 3. To go from sitting on the bed to lying down, bring your feet and knees together, and tighten your core (i.e., your spine and abdomen).

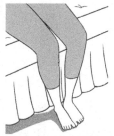

Bring knees and feet together and tighten core.

Step 4. Lean toward the bed with the shoulder you wish to land on as your hands reach for the bed. Keep your core (abdomen and spine) muscles tight and your feet and legs pressed together as gravity lifts your feet up. Then just bend your knees, so your feet land on the bed.

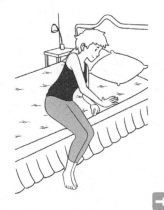

Keep abdomen and spine tight and reach toward bed.

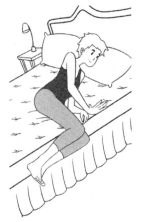 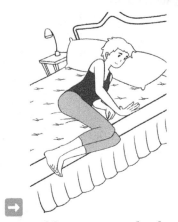

Keep trunk tight as legs rise. **Bend knees onto bed.**

Like a teeter-totter, the weight of your upper body going down will help to lift your feet up. This happens easily if you keep your knees and feet tightly pressed together and your core muscles tight.

Holding your midsection and trunk tight the whole way down allows it to act as a single rigidly supported unit. Otherwise, your upper body will tip away from your hips and create spinal stress.

My best advice is to pretend you are a wooden statue that doesn't bend in the middle at all, and gravity will assist your teeter-totter-like movement with almost no effort on your part.

Part C. Rolling from your side to your back: Steps 5–6.

<u>Step 5.</u> Once your feet have landed on the bed and you are lying securely on your side, then simply roll onto your back. {If you need to, you can give a quick push with your upper (top) hand into the bed and swing your knees and arm up and over to help you land on your back.}

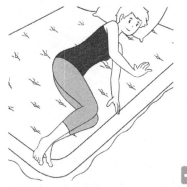

Push your hand into the bed to roll.

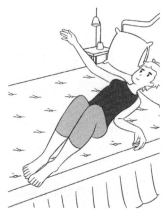

Then swing knees and arm up to finish rolling.

Step 6. Straighten your legs and relax on your back. Or, if you wish to lie on your side, grab your body pillow and roll onto it for a nice nap.

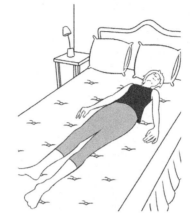

Straighten legs and relax.

OR

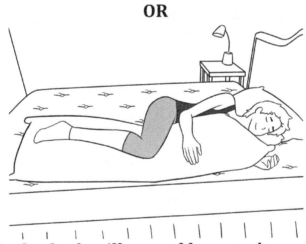

Grab a body pillow and have a nice nap.

Chapter 8

Safe Ways to Get Out of Bed

Part A. Rolling from your back to the edge of the bed.

<u>Step 1.</u> Before rolling onto your side:

To prevent falling off the bed, check to ensure that you are not on, or too close to, the edge of the bed before you roll. You need to secure enough space to accommodate the size of your body before you roll. If you are close to the edge, move over toward the center of the bed. To do this, bend both of your knees and plant your feet flat into the bed as you lift your buttocks up in the air and swing your body away from the edge that you will be rolling toward. Then, slide your shoulders in the same direction, so you line up straight in the bed, a little farther from the edge than you were before.

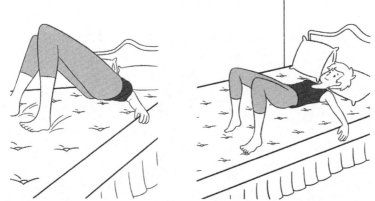

Lift buttocks up and swing your body away from the edge.

How to Roll to the Left

To roll to the **left,** straighten the left leg, bend the right knee, and stick your right arm up toward the ceiling above your heart with the right shoulder at 90 degrees from your chest. From that position, reach your right arm and right knee across your body toward the left edge of the bed, and your body should easily roll onto your left side. **To roll** to the **right** side, do the reverse.

To roll from your back to your side:

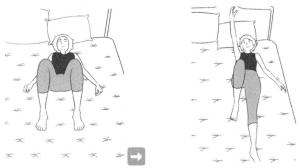

Raise your inside arm and knee.

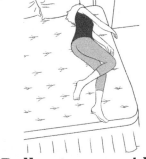

Roll onto your side.

Step 2. Properly position yourself on the edge of the bed.

Once you are on your side, bend your hips and knees (with one leg completely on top of the other), and bring your ankles to the edge of the bed. Place your top hand, palm down on the bed or couch, to a space between your head and the elbow of your other arm that is resting on the bed.

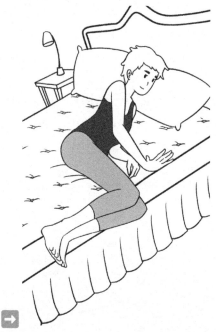

Position feet at the edge of the bed.

Part B. Rising from side-lying to sitting: Steps 3–4.

<u>Step 3.</u> Tighten your core and keep your back rigid and straight.

To prevent back strain and torquing while getting up, tighten your abdomen and back muscles as if you are a rigid wooden board, and keep it tight and straight until you are completely upright. Fully engaging your core in this way allows gravity to assist you in getting up. A floppy core puts your spine at risk for injury and can exacerbate a bulging disk, so be especially mindful of this step. Please note, although some people mistakenly refer to your abdominal muscles as your "core," it is actually your entire trunk, including your abdomen, sides, and back, that collectively make up your core. Just like the core of the apple, it goes all the way around. 😀

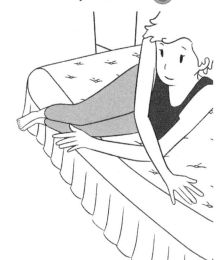

Keep core tight as you push up.

Step 4. Push yourself up to a sitting position.

Press the palm of your top hand into the bed at the very same moment that you let your ankles drop off the side of the bed, as if your palm pushed your ankles off. Then, quickly transfer the power of your push (from the palm of your top arm) to the elbow, then the forearm and hand of your lower (other) arm as you roll up to a sitting position.

The weight of your legs dropping off the bed, with your rigid back, should help lift the weight of your upper body up off the bed effortlessly.

Tighten your core and push into the bed.

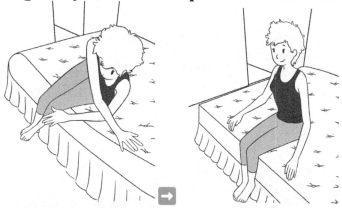

Shift weight to opposite elbow as legs drop and sit up.

Note: As you can see, getting up out of bed requires several steps and synchronized position shifts—none of which entail doing a sit-up!! Sit-ups can round your spine and bulge your discs, so beware! 😉

Another option: Some people find it easier to push their upper hand palm into the lower fist to help press the bent, lower elbow into the bed, while also simultaneously dropping their feet off the bed. They find this helps their leverage and lifts the body up to sitting with less effort.

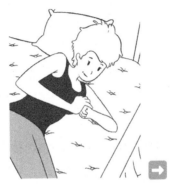

Press into the bed using the lower elbow.

When using this alternative method, the pushing power comes from the upper arm. If this is still difficult, bring your elbow against your belly and try again.

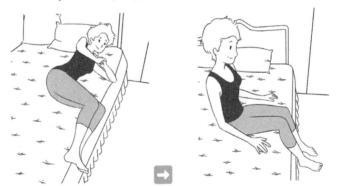

Keep core tight and press into the bed as legs drop.

Part C. Rising from sitting to standing (steps 5-6):

<u>Step 5.</u> Slide your buttocks to the edge.

To rise from a sitting to a standing position, it is important to first come to the edge of the chair, bed, couch, or any other surface you are sitting on. This optimizes your body mechanics by bringing your buttocks more directly over your feet, thus reducing the amount of forward bending necessary to lift yourself up to a standing position.

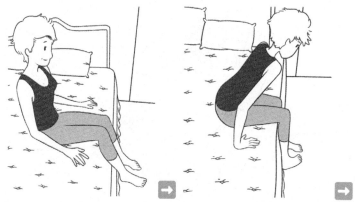

Start from sitting on bed.   Slide buttocks forward.

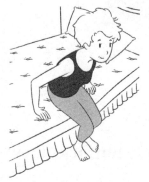

Come to the edge of the bed.

If it is hard to slide your whole bottom forward on a bed, try pushing one side forward at a time, or you can wiggle from side to side as you lean and scooch forward incrementally. If you are in a chair, place both hands on the armrests and press your head and upper back into the back of the chair, and your buttocks should easily slide forward.

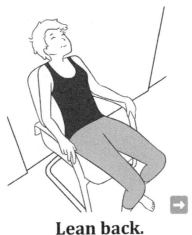

Lean back.

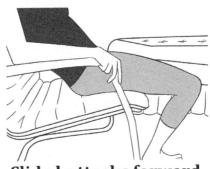

Slide buttocks forward.

Step 6. Push yourself up from sitting to a standing position using your legs with some arm assist, as needed.

Your feet should be approximately hip-width apart, and your hands should be on the armrests of the chair if available, otherwise on the bed or seat on either side of your hips. Your knees and elbows will straighten as you push down with them. Your back should remain straight and upright or slightly forward bent at the hips.

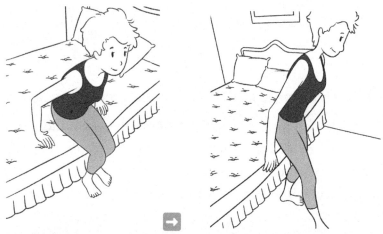

Push with arms and lift with legs to come to stand.

When You Stand: Your head and ribs should lift more up than forward as you straighten and extend your elbows and push down with your hands. Your back should remain well-supported and fairly straight as you rise, using the power in your legs and arms and NOT your back.

In some cases, it can be helpful to have one foot slightly in front of the other. Your back foot can be flat, or on the ball of your foot. You can imagine you are a runner pushing up and out of the starting blocks at the beginning of a race.

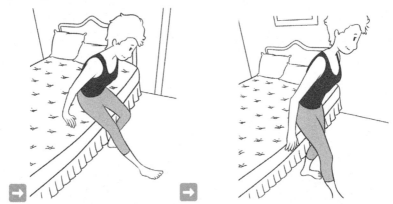

Push with arms and lift with legs to come to stand.

Note: If you have pain or weakness in one leg, definitely put that leg a little forward of the other leg to ease the stress on it. Then using your arms and back leg, push yourself forward and up. You can do this when rising from a bed or a chair.

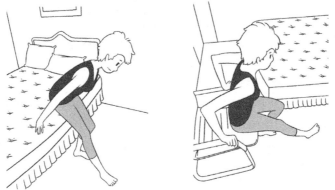

Place weak leg in front.

Summary: Safe Transfers Into and Out of Bed

Getting Into Bed Safely

A. Going from standing to sitting (step 1-2):
> **Step 1.** Touch the bed with both legs.
> **Step 2.** Reach back and sit.

B. Reclining from sitting to side-lying (steps 3-4):
> **Step 3.** Bring feet together and tighten core.
> **Step 4.** Reach, tighten, tip, let gravity help.

C. Rolling from your side to your back (steps 5-6):
> **Step 5.** Swing legs and roll onto your back.
> **Step 6.** Straighten legs and relax.

Getting Out of Bed Safely

A. Rolling from your back to the edge of a bed (steps 1-2):
> **Step 1.** Roll onto your side.
> **Step 2.** Properly position yourself on the edge of the bed.

B. Rising from side-lying to sitting (steps 3-4):
> **Step 3.** Tighten your abdomen and back muscles to keep your core rigid and straight.
> **Step 4.** Push yourself up to a sitting position.

C. Rising from sitting to standing (steps 5-6):
> **Step 5.** Slide your buttocks to the edge of the bed or chair.
> **Step 6.** Push yourself up to a standing position using your legs with some arm assist, as needed.

Chapter 9

Reflux

Reflux is a common problem these days. It can be the result of eating too much, eating too late at night, or eating the wrong foods. It tends to get worse when we lie down in bed at night. It can be intermittent, or it can become a chronic structural problem. It is especially problematic when the stomach pushes itself through the hiatus (opening) between the stomach and the esophagus and gets stuck. This prevents the valve between them from closing properly and allows the acids of the stomach content to erupt upward into the esophagus and throat. It is very unpleasant and can cause symptoms of abdominal pain, chest pain, shortness of breath, and chronic coughing. Since it often mimics the symptoms of a heart attack, many unsuspecting sufferers land in the hospital ER in a panic, only to be diagnosed with a "hiatal hernia."

Reflux Management

Reflux Solution #1: Manage the quantity and quality of the food you eat.

Being aware of what type of foods irritate you, limiting how much food you eat at a time, and being mindful of when you eat can all be very helpful in preventing another attack. Eating and drinking right before bedtime increases the risk of reflux.

Taking digestive enzymes and probiotics with your meals is usually extremely helpful for better digestion and reducing stomach gas buildup. These include over-the-counter type supplements with protease to help digest protein, lipase for fats, and amylase for starches.

Many medical doctors prescribe antacid medication to reduce the amount of acid in your stomach, and though these medications may help reduce your acute symptoms, be careful. Many antacid medications can lead to osteoporosis as a side effect. Also, keep in mind that we need acid in our stomach to digest our foods properly, especially for the proteins we eat.

There are many books on these subjects. The book that I love is titled "*Fit for Life*" by Harvey and Marilyn Diamond.[1] It talks about proper food combining at meals based on the particular digestive chemicals required to break down that particular food. For example, starches like breads, rice, and potatoes require alkaline digestive chemicals to break them down into a more useable form. Proteins like meat, fish, and cheese require acidic digestive chemicals to properly break down the large protein molecules into smaller, more useable amino acids. The book describes in explicit detail how the alkaline and acidic chemicals can work against each other by diminishing the effectiveness of the other so that neither food group can be properly digested in the presence of the other.

---

[1] Harvey Diamond and Marilyn Diamond, *Fit for Life:* (Grand Central Publishing, 1987).

The book presents a wonderful and very detailed explanation of what foods can be eaten together for optimum digestion and which foods should never be eaten together. I highly recommend this book.

Reflux Solution #2: Let gravity assist you by wedging up the head of your bed. Simply place a two-inch brick under the legs that support the head of the bed to create a gentle upward slant to your bed. This creates a gradual incline that elevates your head safely, and it won't kink your neck like placing a bunch of pillows under your head. This position can also help people with mild vertigo and heart issues.

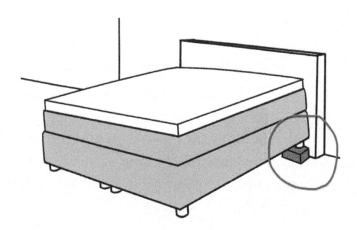

If the brick doesn't wedge you up enough, then you can also slip a large pillow under the head portion of the mattress—between the mattress and the box spring.

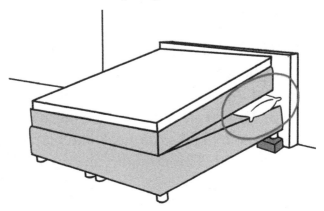

This will raise the head of the bed up a little more and give you a nice 30-degree angle of the whole bed without having to crunch your neck forward on a stack of pillows to elevate your head.

Note: Angling the bed up like this allows gravity to help keep the fluids in your stomach down where they belong, making them less likely to ooze up into your esophagus and throat. I find this position more comfortable than trying to sleep sitting up in a chair. Plus, it is better for your neck and back to be able to stretch out and relax while you sleep.

Chapter 10

Sleeping with Respiratory Issues

Those who have a cold or flu, sinus or lung congestion, or a condition with fluid around the heart generally also find it more comfortable to sleep in a semi-reclined position instead of lying flat. Trying to prop a bunch of pillows under your head and neck is not an ideal solution here either. Bending the head forward and crunching the front of the neck too far may even make the situation worse by kinking the airway in the neck instead of opening it.

A forward bent head position tips the fronts of the neck vertebrae together to create a wedge that can push the disc (located between the vertebra) backward toward the spinal cord. This can cause pain and restrict proper nerve flow to the diaphragm, lungs, and heart.

Therefore, as described in the reflux chapter, I recommend wedging the bed and mattress instead of using several pillows. Have someone place a 2-inch brick or wooden board under the legs that support the head of the bed. It will tip the bed up at an angle, like a tilt table. Then place a wedge pillow or even a fat couch pillow under the mattress to create a more dramatic angle. You may need to modify the size of the brick and wedge pillow depending on the severity of your respiratory condition at the time.

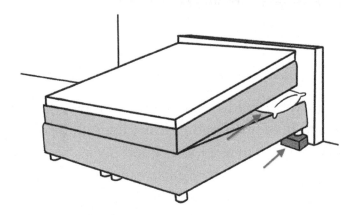

Then if this is not enough, consider purchasing a sturdy, triangular-shaped wedge pillow that starts at your buttocks and incrementally lifts your back and head without bending your neck into a kink.

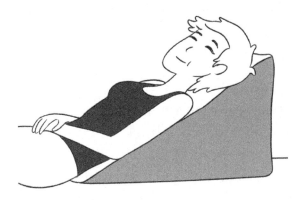

If your condition is more chronic, consider investing in a hand-controlled bed that raises the head of the mattress to your comfort level.

Chapter 11

Wrist Curling and Carpal Tunnel

Many of my patients complain about numbness and tingling in their hands from "carpal tunnel" problems involving compression of the median nerve. The median nerve runs between the carpal bones of the wrist and the thick transverse carpal ligament that bridges over the top of the bones. This ligament creates a tunnel for the nerve and tendons of the hand and fingers to traverse. The medical solution for carpal tunnel is surgical removal of the overlaying transverse carpal ligament. This surgery usually helps in the short term, but it can end up creating scar tissue that recreates the same problem down the road.

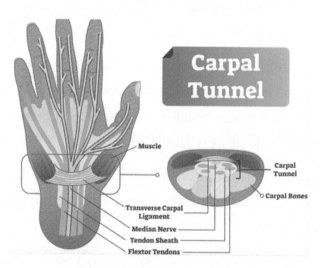

Instead of surgery, a chiropractor would typically adjust the position of the bones of the wrist to provide more room for the nerve to move around under the ligament.

Stretching exercises and manual therapy to lengthen the over-tight flexor muscles of the forearm can also help. In my experience, to maintain the successes gained by manual therapy, it is extremely important for the patient to wear a carpal tunnel brace while sleeping to prevent their hand and palm from curling toward their wrist.

Curling of the fingers and wrist occurs when our well-used and stronger flexor muscles of the palm and forearm overpower the less-used extensor muscles on the back of the hand and forearm.

When we relax during sleep, the imbalance in muscle tone causes the wrist to curl down into a flexed position. Unfortunately, this flexed position of the wrist will cause compression of the median nerve and aggravates the symptoms of carpal tunnel numbness, tingling, pain, and weakness.

Properly bracing the wrist while you sleep prevents this curling and helps decrease the inflammation caused by prolonged pressure. Wearing the brace protects the median nerve from compression so it can rest and heal.

To help you to better understand the mechanics of the median nerve injury in carpal tunnel syndrome, think about a carpet that has furniture on it.

When you move the furniture off of it, you will see that the carpet is indented. If you leave the furniture off the carpet long enough, it will usually puff back up.

The same thing happens in the wrist, where the nerve has been pinched in the carpal tunnel all night. When you first wake up, it's very tingly, prickly, numb, and sometimes painful and weak, but as the day goes on, the nerve starts to heal, and the compressed area begins to decompress. When that happens, the related numbness, tingling, and other symptoms can also start to improve.

If you don't use a splint at night, the nerve will get compressed again from your curled wrist position, and the syndrome begins again. The longer this goes on, the longer it will take for the nerve to recover, and at some point in the future, permanent damage is possible.

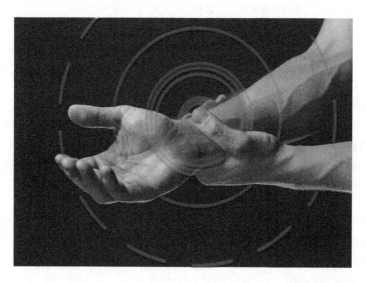

Curling the Wrist While You Sleep

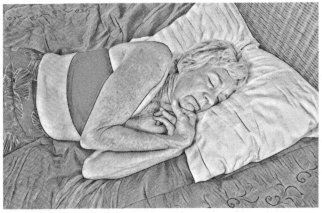

This causes numbness, tingling, and pain and compresses the median nerve.

Wrist Solutions

Wrist Solution #1: Wear a carpal tunnel splint at night while you sleep that extends at least three inches up your forearm and prevents you from bending your wrist. Although there are many carpal tunnel splints on the market, my personal favorite splint is the adjustable "Futuro night wrist brace" by 3M.[2]

This splint is breathable and has a soft pillow in the palm that is very soothing. It is easy to adjust with Velcro straps, and it fits wrists measuring 5.25–9 inches. You can find it on Amazon, and the cost is around $25–32 per splint.

---

[2] "FUTURO-48462 Night Wrist Support SIOC, Helps Provide Nighttime Relief of Carpel Tunnel Symptoms, Breathable, One Size ." Amazon. Amazon.com. Accessed January 17, 2022.

Note: Be sure the brace is comfortable and fairly loose, so you don't constrict the circulation and add to the numbness. The goal of the splint is just to keep you from folding your wrist too far. A small amount of wrist movement within the brace is okay.

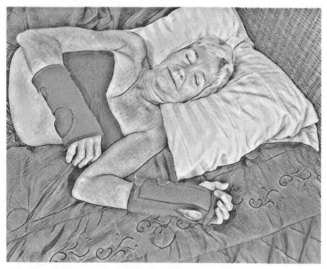

Night wrist supports are breathable and comfortable but will stabilize your wrists at night.

Wrist Solution #2: Take vitamin B6 and B12 to help reduce inflammation, rebuild the nerve's protective myelin sheath, and improve nerve function in the wrist and hand.

Chapter 12

Beds, Mattresses, and Perfect Pillows

? ? ?

Patients frequently ask me about beds, mattresses, and pillows. What are the best ones, how firm, how thick, what type should I get? These are difficult questions for me to answer because everyone is so different in their body type, needs, and preferences.

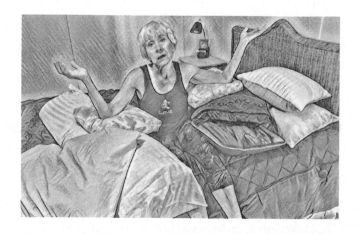

1. Bed Mattresses: The best bed for you is the one that makes you feel comfortable when you are awake and lying on it, and one where you still feel good when you wake up after sleeping on it all night.

Typically, it is a good idea to replace your bed at least every 10–15 years because beds can break down and get lumpy, or get ruts or indentations where your body has compressed the bed over time.

It can also develop a buildup of microorganisms and bacteria that could potentially affect your health if not protected properly by a hypoallergenic mattress cover.

It is important to find a bed that is supportive but not too firm. Otherwise, it can cause pressure on your hip and shoulder joints when sleeping on your side. You also want a bed that is soft enough to give cushion to your joints but not so soft that you lose the support needed to protect your spinal alignment. Now you see why it is a difficult task to find the best of both worlds, especially for people of different body types who share the same bed.

a. Tempurpedic Beds: I would also like to discuss the differences that I experienced between memory foam and Tempurpedic beds. Tempurpedic mattresses are body temperature controlled, so when your warm body lies on the bed, the bed softens and cushions around your body parts. However, when you want to roll over, you must first lift up and out of the gully your body has made and sunk into before you will be able to turn.

If the room is cold, the bed will be firmer, making it even more difficult to turn. As a result, it will take more time for you to melt back into the Tempurpedic bed comfortably and for your previous indentations to come back to neutral.

b. Memory Foam Beds: Memory foam beds, on the other hand, are pressure-sensitive, so when you lie on them, the foam will indent to fit your body's boney prominences, but as soon as you lift up, the indentations will disappear, and the place you roll to will immediately respond to your pressure without having to warm it up. For this reason, I personally much prefer the memory foam-type beds to the Tempurpedic mattresses.

c. Push-Button Adjustable Beds: Patients also ask me about the push-button adjustable beds that have several functions such as sitting you up, lowering you down, raising the legs, or getting firmer and softer than the other side so both people in the bed can be comfortable even though their body types are different. I think the concept is great and probably the way of the future, but they tend to be quite expensive and out of many people's budget. That being said, the people I know who have invested in these beds tend to be very happy with them.

Bed Solutions

1. The Best Bed: The best bed for you is the one you try out in the store that feels good to you and whoever shares the bed with you. Be sure it has a multi-month guarantee of a full refund. That way, you have options if, after you get it home and actually sleep in it for several nights, it no longer feels so good.

2. Memory Foam Mat: If you currently have a bed that is causing you discomfort because it is too firm or lumpy, or if you have a Tempurpedic bed that is hard for you to turn on, you can purchase a memory foam mat for your bed. They come in various sizes. Simply lay it on top of the bed (under the mattress pad), and it will provide supportive comfort at a much lower cost than buying a memory foam bed, especially if one is out of your budget. If you are currently still researching the best bed for you, a memory foam mat can also work as a temporary fix until you can find a more comfortable bed than the one you may currently have.

Please note: Though the memory foam mats are comfortable, they do not last as long or provide as much support as a memory foam bed, and they are quite unpleasantly stinky from the plastic shrink wrap when you first get them. Therefore, they will need to "off-gas" for a week or so in a guest room or basement before you use them.

The best ones come with their own cover to protect the memory foam from getting torn or frayed. They fit very tightly over the foam and often require two people to get the cover back on after washing it. I do not recommend using memory foam without a protective cover.

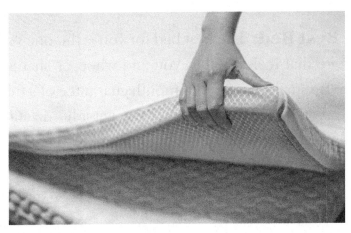

Memory Foam Solution

My husband and I travel with a two-inch-thick queen-size memory foam mat in our van so we can sleep anywhere, from the floor to a lumpy bed or a pull-out couch. We just place our mat on top of any surface we wish to sleep on, and it provides comfort and support for us both. I know it has saved my back and joints many times.

3. Perfect Pillows: Finding the "perfect pillow" can be a very difficult and frustrating process. There are numerous varieties, shapes, and sizes. Some have prefab depressions to fit your head so you get support, whether you are on your back or your side. Some even have a neck roll built into them. Some are squishy like feathers, and others are firm foam or bean-filled. I am convinced that there is a pillow out there for everyone, but I don't believe there is any one pillow that is good for everyone.

Those with delicate and smaller necks need a smaller, thinner pillow under their head than a larger individual. I have searched my whole life to find the perfect pillow for myself, but I admit, it may or may not work as well for someone else. Therefore, I suggest people use pillows that fit their particular body structure. When side sleeping, use a pillow under the head that takes up the width of your shoulder, and when on your back, try using a very thin pillow or none at all.

If you have allergies, asthma, or sinus issues, I recommend you try to avoid feather pillows, as feathers and down can be irritants for these conditions.

I also recommend that you get a very good hypoallergenic pillow cover to protect yourself from any chemicals, allergens, or microscopic organisms that could be in your pillow. These zip-on covers also protect the pillow from anything your body might leak onto its surface, such as saliva, blood, or mucus. They can be more easily removed and washed than the pillow itself, and a proper protective cover (in addition to your pillowcase) will extend the life of your beloved comfy pillow.

Neck Pillow Solution

My personal preference for a neck pillow is the Brookstone Store's "Better than Down Pillow."[3] I like it because it is hypoallergenic—i.e., no feathers to aggravate allergies and asthma—but it is squishy like a feather pillow, and it holds its shape after you fluff it under your neck. Unfortunately, I am not sure Brookstone still makes it. 😳

---

3 "'Better than Down Pillow.,'" "Better than Down Pillow." (Brookstone.com), accessed January 17, 2022, www.brookstone.com.

4. Body pillows: In addition to a pillow under your neck, you should have something that mimics a body pillow on either side of your body to catch and support your top leg and arm when you sleep on your side. The pillow should be beside your bottom leg, NOT between your legs.

You don't need to spend $90 on a store-bought body pillow. You can easily make your own.

A good body pillow should match the height of your hips. If it does, it will allow your top leg and arm to remain parallel with the bed and level when they are on the pillow. It will also allow your other leg, the one still resting on the bed, to completely stretch out as straight as it wants.

Your bottom leg should be beside and behind the pillow, NOT underneath it.

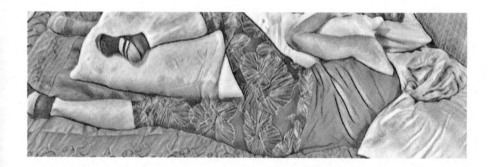

Body Pillow Solution

My personal solution for a body pillow is to make your own using two spare pillows, a towel, a fleece (or cotton blanket), and two soft pillowcases. For the summertime, cover your roll with a sheet or two king-size pillowcases, so it's not too warm for those hot summer nights.

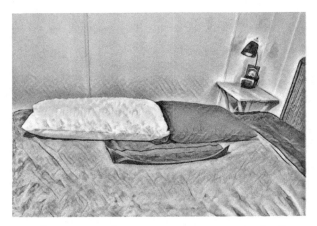

Continue to the next chapter to see exactly how to make your own body pillow.

Chapter 13

How to Make a Body Pillow

It would be nice if you could find a body-length pillow that just happens to be the right thickness for your hips and body length at an affordable price, but it is not necessary. Making your own custom-sized body pillow is very easy and often more comfortable than the expensive store-bought models.

First, get a sense of the distance between your hips. Wide hips need a larger diameter pillow, and narrow hips need a smaller, less puffy pillow. The goal is to place your top leg on the pillow so that your thigh is parallel to the bed without tilting up or down at the knee or the ankle. The length of the pillow also depends on your personal body type and height. The final length of the pillow should extend from your ankle to your upper chest.

Next, obtain two standard or king-size pillows. Check to see if you have some old pillows that are too large for your head and too short to be body pillow length by themselves. Grab two of these pillows, a large bath or beach towel, a large blanket, and two pillowcases, and make your own body pillow.

If you don't have pillows, buy two inexpensive standard or king pillows and proceed with the directions below. It will still be less expensive than buying a body pillow.

Steps:

1. Spread the blanket out on the bed.

2. Lay one end of an unfolded towel onto the left edge of the blanket (about halfway between the top and bottom of the blanket). The towel dimensions (left to right) should be longer than its width (top to bottom).

3. Place the two pillows end to end on the center of the towel.

4. Wrap the towel around the junction point of the two pillows to help secure them together.

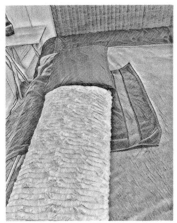 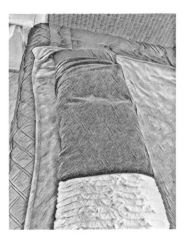

Steps 1, 2, and 3.   Step 4.

5. Roll the blanket around the bundle of pillows secured with the towel.

6. Keep rolling the blanket like a sleeping bag until either there is no more blanket, or the height of the roll is proportional to your hip width.

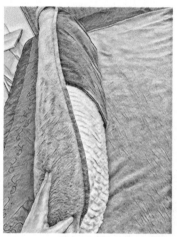
Step 5.

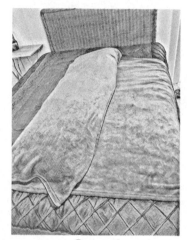
Step 6.

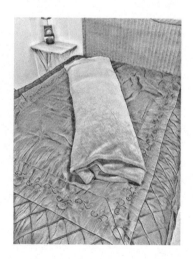

7. Secure the blanket ends with a pillowcase on each end of the blanket roll. If you have too much blanket for your pelvis height, just fold or scrunch it up next to your roll and then add the pillowcases.

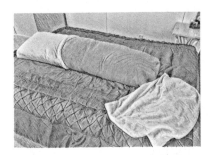

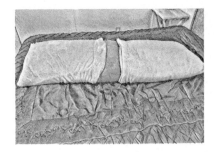

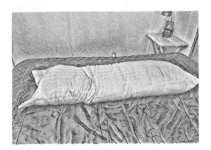

Step 7.

8. Try it out for pillow length and diameter to be sure it is comfortable and proportional to your hip width and body length.

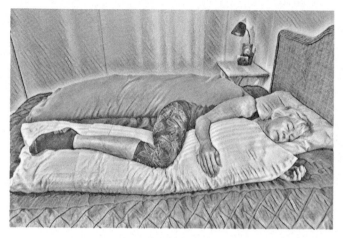

Step 8.

9. If you need a smaller diameter pillow, you can use a smaller blanket or even a sheet. If you need a larger diameter pillow, wrap another blanket around it. It all depends on the thickness of your pillows in relation to your own body size. In the end, it will be worth the effort.

Chapter 14

Conclusion

Sleeping is something we all do. Unfortunately, the way we sleep can sabotage our spinal alignment and lead to pain and dysfunction that interfere with our daily lives—no matter how good our daytime habits may be.

I cannot over-emphasize the importance of good posture and proper positioning during sleep. Not only will it improve the quality of your sleep, it will help you avoid the nagging pain, stiffness, and dysfunction that so many people experience upon awakening. Proper positioning and good pillow support also help protect the nerve and blood flow to your brain from being compromised by the spinal twisting and torquing that can otherwise happen while you sleep.

Remember to download your free digital copy of *"How to make your own body pillow"* and the summary of *"How to transfer in and out of bed safely"* at KMFbooks.com.

May your sleep be biomechanically sound, comfortable, and healing. And may you wake up refreshed, limber, and pain-free with enough energy, strength, and flexibility to carry you through your whole day. 🙂

Thank You For Reading *Solutions for Better Sleep!*

This is the first book of my *Preventing Spinal Sabotage: Mayhem, Myths and Management Series*. If you found this book beneficial, help spread the word on Facebook (or with an Amazon review), and feel free to share your book and the free downloads with your family and friends.

All my books are meant to empower you, my patients and readers, with a variety of simple and effective tools to improve posture, body mechanics, and spinal alignment. You will gain a better understanding of your spine, how it works and how to protect it. These well-illustrated (and slightly whimsical) books will help relieve pain and improve flexibility so you can enjoy a healthier, happier, more energetic life.

For the latest information on my upcoming books, to leave me a message, or to get your free downloads, check out my website at KMFbooks.com. To leave a review, visit amazon.com.

☺ Acknowledgments ☺

I would like to thank my husband, parents, and my three beta readers, Julie, Carol, and Barbara, for reading and critiquing my book in its early phases. Special thanks to my model, June Evans. Thank you to my two talented Upwork artists, Josiah Branal, who did the line drawings, and Viktoriia Davidova, who drew the picture on the book cover.

Very special thanks to Jeannie Culbertson for her kind words of reassurance and encouragement and her guidance and support on editing and formatting. Thanks to my fellow students and coaches at SPS and to all who have enjoyed reading and reviewing my book.

Lastly, and most importantly, I would like to say a very special thanks to all of my beloved patients who, over the years, inspired me to write this all down. I wrote this book for their benefit and for all those in pain or in need of better sleeping habits.

About the Author

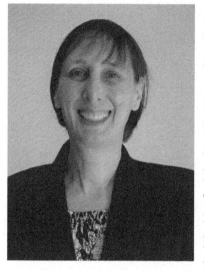

Dr. Kathleen M. Favaloro is a Chiropractor, Physical Therapist, grandmother, and a 4th Degree Black belt Master in Taekwondo. She has over 40 years in the healing field and over 20 years in the martial arts. She has a passion for helping people to achieve their potential and enjoys teaching Taekwondo as much as she enjoys working with patients.

In 2020, she combined her talents to help produce a one-hour educational video for seniors called *Self-defense and Safety Awareness for Seniors.* It is available at 3seniors.com.

Her first two children's books in her Tommy Book Series, *"Tommy Takes Taekwondo"* and *"Bullies, Friends, and Taekwondo,"* will soon be available on Amazon. Check KMFbooks.com for details. These books emphasize Taekwondo philosophy as they follow a timid young boy's journey into Taekwondo, where he learns confidence and ways to handle his challenges—even with bullies, in unique, non-violent ways.

Dr. Favaloro remains committed to finishing her three-volume book titled *"Preventing Spinal Sabotage: Mayhem, Myths, and Management."* It is a somewhat whimsical and educational guide to taking care of your spine.

Made in the USA
Coppell, TX
17 April 2023

15720894R00056